Instructor's Manual and Test Bank for

Calculation of Drug Dosages

Seventh Edition

Sheila J. Ogden, MSN, RN

Orthopaedics Program Director
Clarian Health Partners
Indianapolis, Indiana

Linda K. Fluharty, MSN, RN

Associate Professor
ASN Program
Ivy Tech State College
Indianapolis, Indiana

 **Mosby**

An Affiliate of Elsevier Science

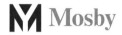

An Affiliate of Elsevier Science

11830 Westline Industrial Drive
St. Louis, Missouri 63146

INSTRUCTOR'S MANUAL AND TEST BANK   ISBN 0-323-02421-1
FOR CALCULATION OF DRUG DOSAGES, SEVENTH EDITION

Copyright © 2003, Mosby, Inc. All rights reserved.

Executive Vice President, Nursing and Health Professions: Sally Schrefer
Acquisitions Editor: Yvonne Alexopoulos
Associate Developmental Editor: Danielle M. Frazier
Publishing Services Manager: Catherine Jackson
Project Manager: Clay S. Broeker
Design Manager: Teresa Breckwoldt

Printed in the United States of America

Last digit is the print number: 9 8 7 6 5 4 3 2 1

PREFACE

The *Instructor's Manual and Test Bank for Calculation of Drug Dosages* was written to provide suggestions for using the work text. Part I is composed of suggested class schedules. One schedule is provided for a 16-week course, and a second schedule is provided for a 9-week course.

Part II provides teaching strategies and tips plus handouts for areas of content covered within the work text. The strategies include suggestions for timing of quizzes, discussion points for each class, areas that have proved difficult for some students in the past, assignments for each class, and additional examples for demonstration.

Part III includes originals for overhead transparencies that can be made for use in the classroom.

Part IV provides a test bank of additional problems not currently found in the student's work text. Problems covering the review of mathematics areas plus specific calculations of the wide variety of drug dosages included in the work text are provided. The test bank may be used for "pop" quizzes, for additional problems if a student is having difficulty with a particular concept, or for the development of the instructor's unique comprehensive examination. The answers for all test bank questions are included in Part V.

We hope the addition of this resource is helpful to instructors as they teach and facilitate the student's mastery of the content of *Calculation of Drug Dosages*.

Sheila J. Ogden, MSN, RN
Linda K. Fluharty, MSN, RN

CONTENTS

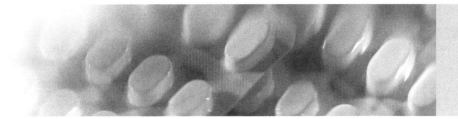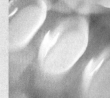

I

Suggested Class Schedules

16-WEEK COURSE

WEEK 1   Chapters 1 and 2: Fractions and Decimals

WEEK 2   Chapters 3 and 4: Percents and Ratios

WEEK 3   Chapter 5: Proportions

WEEK 4   Final Math Review

WEEK 5   Chapters 6 and 7: Metric, Apothecary, and Household Measurements

WEEK 6   Chapter 8: Equivalents between Apothecary and Metric Measurements

WEEK 7   Chapter 9: Interpretation of the Physician's Orders

WEEK 8   Chapter 10: How to Read Drug Labels

WEEK 9   Chapters 11 and 12: Dimensional Analysis and Oral Dosages

WEEK 10 Chapter 13: Parenteral Dosages

WEEK 11 Chapter 14: Dosages Measured in Units

WEEK 12 Chapter 15: Intravenous Flow Rates

WEEK 13 Chapter 16: Critical Care IV Flow Rates

WEEK 14 Chapter 17: Pediatric Dosages

WEEK 15 Chapters 18, 19, and 20 and Case Studies

WEEK 16 Final Examination and Laboratory Check Off Suggested

9-WEEK COURSE

WEEK 1   Chapters 1 through 5: Fractions, Decimals, Percents, Ratios, and Proportions

WEEK 2   Chapters 6 through 8: Metric, Apothecary, and Household Measurements, and Equivalents

WEEK 3   Chapters 9 and 10: Interpretation of the Physician's Orders and How to Read Drug Labels

WEEK 4   Chapters 11 and 12: Dimensional Analysis and Oral Dosages

WEEK 5   Chapters 13 and 14: Parenteral Dosages and Dosages Measured in Units

WEEK 6   Chapter 15: Intravenous Flow Rates

WEEK 7   Chapter 16: Critical Care IV Flow Rates

WEEK 8   Chapter 17: Pediatric Dosages

WEEK 9   Chapters 18, 19, and 20; Case Studies and Review

1

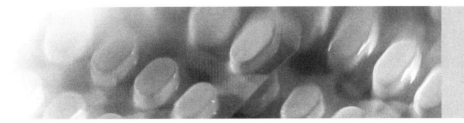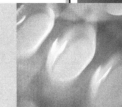

II

Chapter Teaching Strategies and Tips

WEEK 1

A. Complete an introduction to the class. Discuss class schedule and grading, as well as student and teacher responsibilities.
B. Administer the "Mathematics Pretest."
C. Briefly discuss the content of Chapter 1, "Fractions."
   Work various problems in class that involve complex fractions.
   Emphasize that the denominator of a whole number is always "1."
D. Briefly discuss the content of Chapter 2, "Decimals."
   Work multiplication and division problems in class.
   Practice rounding with the students.
   Discuss multiplying and dividing shortcuts when the multiplier and divisor are 10 or 0.1 and multiples of each.
E. *Assignment*: 1. Fraction Work Sheet
   2. Fraction Posttest 1
   3. Decimal Work Sheet
   4. Decimal Posttest 1
F. Allow time in class to begin assignments and to answer questions.

WEEK 2

A. Administer the quiz that covers fractions and decimals.
   Use either the Pretest or the Posttest 2 questions.
B. Briefly discuss the content of Chapter 3, "Percents."
   Emphasize that the denominator of a percent is always 100.
   Specifically work problems that involve what the percent of one number is of another, and work problems that find a given percent of a number. These concepts are usually the hardest for the student. Relate a percent of a number to shopping where the sale price is "20%" off the original price.
C. Briefly discuss the content of Chapter 4, "Ratios."
   If students have mastered the content of the previous chapters, ratios are usually an easy concept for them to understand.
D. *Assignment:* 1. Percent Work Sheet
   2. Percent Posttest 1
   3. Ratio Work Sheet
   4. Ratio Posttest 1
E. Allow time in class to begin assignments and to answer questions.

3

Copyright © 2003 Mosby, Inc. All rights reserved.

WEEK 3

A. Administer the quiz that covers percents and ratios.
   Use either the Pretest or the Posttest 2 questions.
B. Briefly discuss the content of Chapter 5, "Proportions."
   Specifically work each type of proportion problem in class. This exercise also serves as a review for previous week's content.
C. *Assignment*: 1. Proportion Work Sheet
                     2. Proportion Posttest 1
D. Allow time in class to begin assignments and to answer questions.

WEEK 4

A. Discuss questions or concerns of students from Chapters 1 through 5.
B. Administer the Mathematics Posttest.

WEEK 5

A. Briefly discuss the content of Chapter 6, "Metric and Household Measurements."
B. Work several problems in class.
C. *Assignment:* 1. Metric and Household Work Sheet
                     2. Metric and Household Posttest 1
D. Briefly discuss the content of Chapter 7, "Apothecary and Household Measurement."
E. *Assignment:* 1. Apothecary and Household Work Sheet
                     2. Apothecary and Household Posttest 1
F. Allow time in class to begin assignments and to answer questions.

WEEK 6

A. Administer the quiz that covers metric, apothecary and household measurements. Use either the Pretest or Posttest 2 questions.
B. Briefly discuss the content of Chapter 8, "Equivalents between Apothecary and Metric Measurements."
C. Work and discuss each type of problem.
D. *Assignment:* 1. Equivalents Work Sheet
                     2. Equivalents Posttest 2
E. Allow time in class to begin assignments and to answer questions.

WEEK 7

A. Administer the quiz that covers equivalents between metric and apothecary measurements and household measurements.
   Use either Pretest or Posttest 2 questions.
B. Briefly discuss the content of Chapter 9, "Interpretation of the Physician's Orders." If the students have clinical experiences, suggest they bring samples of medical administration records to the next class for discussion.
C. *Assignment:* 1. Posttest 1

WEEK 8

A. Briefly discuss the content of Chapter 10, "How to Read Drug Labels."
B. *Assignment:* 1. Posttest 1
               2. Posttest 2
C. Allow time in class to begin assignments and to answer questions.

WEEK 9

A. Administer the quiz that covers parts of drug labels. Choose a variety of labels from the student textbook, and label the various parts in the same format as the Posttest.
B. Briefly discuss the content of Chapter 11, "Dimensional Analysis and the Calculation of Drug Dosages."
C. Briefly discuss the content of Chapter 12, "Oral Dosages." At this time, have students choose the method they prefer when calculating drug dosages. Strongly encourage them to retain the same method throughout the rest of the class rather than change methods.
D. *Assignment:* 1. Oral Dosage Work Sheet
               2. Oral Dosage Posttest 1
E. Allow time in class to begin assignments and to answer questions.

WEEK 10

A. Administer the quiz that covers oral dosages. Use Posttest 2.
B. Briefly discuss the content of Chapter 13, "Parenteral Dosages."
C. *Assignment:* 1. Parenteral Dosage Work Sheet
               2. Parenteral Dosage Posttest 1
D. Allow time in class to begin assignments and to answer questions.

WEEK 11

A. Administer the quiz that covers parenteral dosages. Use Posttest 2.
B. Briefly discuss the content of Chapter 14, "Dosages Measured in Units." Remind students that problems involving units are calculated the same way as they have been calculating problems in the previous two chapters. Review several examples of powdered medications that require constitution, which is always a difficult concept for students.
C. *Assignment:* 1. Dosages Measured in Units Work Sheet
               2. Dosages Measured in Units Posttest 1
D. Allow time in class to begin assignments and to answer questions.

WEEK 12

A. Administer the quiz that covers dosages measured in units. Use Posttest 2.
B. Briefly discuss the content of Chapter 15, "Intravenous Flow Rates."
C. *Assignment:* 1. IV Flow Rate Work Sheet
               2. IV Flow Rate Posttest 1
D. Allow time in class to begin assignments and to answer questions.

WEEK 13

A. Give quiz over intravenous (IV) flow rates. Suggest using Posttest 2 questions.
B. Briefly discuss the content of Chapter 16, "Critical Care IV Flow Rates."
C. *Assignment:* 1. Critical Care Medications Work Sheet
               2. Critical Care Medications Posttest 1
D. Allow time in class to begin assignments and to answer questions.

WEEK 14

A. Administer the quiz that covers IV administration of critical care medications. Use Posttest 2.
B. Briefly discuss the content of Chapter 17, "Pediatric Dosages." Review each step of completing a pediatric drug dosage problem when based on weight. In addition, practice on body surface calculations, and use the nomogram for calculations of pediatric medications.
C. *Assignment:* 1. Pediatric Work Sheet
                2. Pediatric Posttest 1
D. Allow time in class to begin assignments and to answer questions.

WEEK 15

A. Administer the quiz that covers pediatric drug calculations.
B. Briefly discuss the content of Chapters 18, 19, and 20.
C. Have students complete case studies in class.
D. *Assignment:* 1. Study for cumulative final examination.

WEEK 16

A. Administer the Final Examination and Laboratory Check Off.
B. Evaluate class performance.

  PART II Chapter Teaching Strategies and Tips

TEACHING TIPS

CHAPTERS 6 and 7

Distribute a copy of the "Systems of Measurement" handout (see page 11) to each student. Discuss the metric, apothecary, and household measurements. Information regarding the unit and milliequivalent system is also added for additional student information, if the instructor desires.

CHAPTER 8

Distribute a copy of the "Equivalents" handout (see page 13) to each student. Review the information contained in the "Conversions Teaching Outline for the Classroom." In addition to the ratio-proportion and algebraic methods for conversions, introduce the conversion factor method, if desired.

 Write a conversion on the board (see the examples on the "Equivalents" handout). The decision to show only the ratio-proportion method may be made, or the algebraic or conversion factor methods may also be illustrated to solve conversion problems.

CHAPTER 12

Write dosage calculation problems on the board, and demonstrate the ratio-proportion method and the following method to solve the problems.

$$\frac{D}{A} \times Q = x$$

Example 1: Order: Acetaminophen 280 mg po q4h prn T > 100.6
      Available: Acetaminophen drops 80 mg/0.8 mL

$$80 \text{ mg} : 0.8 \text{ mL} :: 280 \text{ mg} : x \text{ mL} \qquad \textbf{OR} \qquad \frac{280 \text{ mg}}{80 \text{ mg}} \times 0.8 \text{ mL} = \frac{224}{80} = 2.8 \text{ mL}$$

$$80x = 224$$

$$\frac{80x}{80} = \frac{224}{80}$$

$$x = 2.8 \text{ mL}$$

Example 2: Order: Keflex 375 mg per gastrostomy tube (GT) q6h
Available: Keflex 250 mg/5 mL

$$250 \text{ mg} : 5 \text{ mL} :: 375 \text{ mg} : x \text{ mL} \quad \textbf{\textit{OR}} \quad \frac{375 \text{ mg}}{250 \text{ mg}} \times 5 \text{ mL} = \frac{1875}{250} = 7.5 \text{ mL}$$

$$250x = 1875$$

$$\frac{250x}{250} = \frac{1875}{250}$$

$$x = 7.5 \text{ mL}$$

CHAPTER 13

Write dosage calculation problems on the board and demonstrate both the ratio-proportion method and the following method to solve the problems.

$$\frac{D}{A} \times Q = x$$

As the problems are solved, show different sized syringes that would be appropriate for the amount of medication required (see Transparency Originals 14 and 16 that illustrate syringes).

Example for Parenteral Order: Morphine sulfate 10 mg intramuscularly (IM) q4h prn for pain
Available: Morphine sulfate gr $^{1}/_{4}$ per 1 mL

$$\text{Convert grains to mg: gr } \frac{1}{4} \times 60 \text{ mg} = \frac{60}{4} \text{ mg} = 15 \text{ mg}$$

$$15 \text{ mg} : 1 \text{ mL} :: 10 \text{ mg} : x \text{ mL} \quad \textbf{\textit{OR}} \quad \frac{10 \text{ mg}}{15 \text{ mg}} \times 1 \text{ mL} = 0.66 \text{ or } 0.7 \text{ mL}$$

$$15x = 10$$

$$\frac{15x}{15} = \frac{10}{15}$$

$$x = 0.66 \text{ or } 0.7 \text{ mL}$$

Example for Units Order: Heparin 7500 U SC now
Available: Heparin 20,000 U/1 mL

$$20,000 \text{ U} : 1 \text{ mL} :: 7500 \text{ U} : x \text{ mL} \quad \textbf{\textit{OR}} \quad \frac{7500 \text{ U}}{20,000 \text{ U}} \times 1 \text{ mL} = 0.375 \text{ or } 0.38 \text{ mL}$$

$$20,000x = 7500$$

$$\frac{20,000x}{20,000} = \frac{7500}{20,000}$$

$$x = 0.375 \text{ or } 0.38 \text{ mL}$$

CHAPTER 15

Begin by explaining the different tubing drop factors. Having different IV tubings to show the students would be helpful. After discussing the examples in the text, continue by working the first three problems listed on the work sheet with the students. (The answers can be found in the back of the dosage calculation text.)

CHAPTER 16

After discussing the examples in the text, continue by working the first two problems listed on the work sheet with the students. (The answers can be found in the back of the dosage calculation text.)

SYSTEMS OF MEASUREMENT

Metric System

1. The metric system is used most often for prescriptions and drug labels.
2. This system uses the decimal system. It does not use fractions; for example, 1.5 not $1^1/_2$.
3. If the decimal is less than 1, then a 0 should precede the decimal; for example, 0.8.
4. A drug can be measured by weight, volume, or length within the metric system.
5. When measuring a drug by weight, the gram (g) is the base unit. All other units used to measure a drug by weight are compared with the gram. The kilogram (kg) is 1000 times more than the gram, whereas the milligram (mg) is 1/1000th of a gram. The microgram (mcg) is 1/1,000,000th of a gram. For the visual learner, the following diagram may be helpful to understand how these measurements compare with one another.

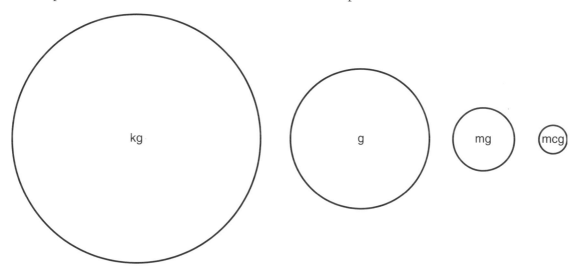

Therefore 1 kg = 1000 g
1 g = 1000 mg
1 mg = 1000 mcg

6. When measuring a drug by volume, the liter (L) is the base unit. A milliliter (mL) is a second unit that is used to measure a drug by volume, and it is compared with the liter. A milliliter is 1/1000th of a liter.

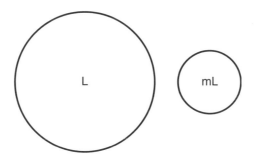

Therefore 1 L = 1000 mL (or cc)

7. When measuring length, the meter (m) is the base unit. The other units used to measure a drug by length are compared with the meter. The centimeter (cm) is 1/100th of a meter, and the millimeter (mm) is 1/1000th of a meter.

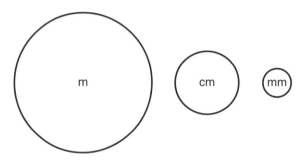

Therefore 1 m = 100 cm
          1 m = 1000 mm

Apothecary System

1. The apothecary system is still used, usually by physicians trained on this system.
2. This system is still used to prescribe some common medications (e.g., aspirin, Tylenol, codeine).
3. The abbreviation or unit symbol precedes the quantity of the medication; for example, gr $^1/_4$.
4. This system uses Roman numerals for amounts ranging from 1 to 10; for example, gr V. It uses fractions for amounts less than 1; for example, gr $^1/_2$.

Household System

1. The household system is commonly used for medications given at home and for pediatric patients.
2. This system uses Arabic numbers; for example, 1 tablespoon.
3. It uses fractions for numbers less than 1; for example, $^1/_4$ teaspoon.

Unit System

1. The unit system is expressed in Arabic numbers, followed by the word unit or international unit (IU).
2. IUs may be used to represent the potency of vitamins and chemicals.
3. Units may be used to prescribe penicillin, heparin, and insulin.
4. A milliunit (mU) is 1/1000th of a unit and is used for medications (e.g., Pitocin).

Milliequivalent System

1. Milliequivalent (mEq) system is expressed in Arabic numbers.
2. A milliequivalent is 1/1000th of a chemical weight.
3. This system is commonly used when prescribing electrolytes, such as calcium, magnesium, and potassium.

HANDOUT Systems of Measurement

EQUIVALENTS

1. The nurse performs conversions when the unit of measurement in the drug order is different from the unit of measurement in the supplied drug. There are three methods from which to choose: ratio-proportion, algebraic, or conversion factor.
2. The text has explanations for both the ratio-proportion and algebraic conversion methods. For the conversion factor, there are two steps. The first step is to identify the appropriate equivalency; the second step involves either multiplying or dividing.

   The general rule is to convert a larger unit of measurement to a smaller unit or a smaller unit of measurement to a larger unit. To convert a unit to a smaller measurement, the health care professional (HCP) should multiply; to convert a unit to a larger measurement, the HCP should divide.

   Example: Find the number of milliliters that are equivalent to 3 tablespoons

   $$3 \text{ T} = \underline{\hspace{1cm}} \text{ mL}$$

   Step 1—Identify the equivalent of 1 T = 15 mL.
   Step 2—The tablespoon is a larger unit than a milliliter because 1 tablespoon is equal to 15 milliliters. Therefore when converting from the larger unit (3 T) to the smaller unit (? mL), multiplication is required. The formula would be:

   $$3 \times 15 = 45, \text{ so } 3 \text{ T} = 45 \text{ mL}$$

3. Write the conversion on the board to illustrate all three methods to the students. After the students have practiced the methods, they can choose the one with which they are most comfortable.

   Example 1: 12 cups = _____ quarts

Ratio-Proportion	Algebraic	Conversion Factor
1 qt : 4 cups :: x qt : 12 cups	$\dfrac{1 \text{ qt}}{4 \text{ cups}} = \dfrac{x \text{ qt}}{12 \text{ cups}}$	Smaller to larger, so you divide
$4x = 12$		1 qt = 4 cups
	$4x = 12$	
$\dfrac{4x}{4} = \dfrac{12}{4}$		12 cups ÷ 4 cups = 3
	$\dfrac{4x}{4} = \dfrac{12}{4}$	
$x = 3$		
	$x = 3$	

   Example 2: 6 feet = _____ inches

1 foot : 12 inches :: 6 feet : x inches	$\dfrac{1 \text{ ft}}{12 \text{ in}} = \dfrac{6 \text{ ft}}{x \text{ in}}$	Larger to smaller, so you multiply
$x = 12 \times 6$		
$x = 72$		1 ft − 12 inches
	$x = 72$	
		6 ft × 12 − 72 inches

Example 3: 500 mL = _____ L

Ratio-Proportion	Algebraic	Conversion Factor

1 L : 1000 mL :: x L : 500 mL

$$\frac{1\text{ L}}{1000\text{ mL}} = \frac{x\text{ L}}{500\text{ mL}}$$

Smaller to larger, so you divide

$1000x = 500$

$$\frac{1\cancel{000}x}{1\cancel{000}} = \frac{500}{1000}$$

$1000x = 500$

$$\frac{1\cancel{000}x}{1\cancel{000}} = \frac{500}{1000}$$

1 L = 1000 mL

$500 \div 1000 = 0.5$

OR

$0.500.$

$x = \frac{1}{2}$ or 0.5

$x = \frac{1}{2}$ or 0.5

When dividing in the metric system—move the decimal point to the left

Example 4: 0.015 g = _____ mg

g : 1000 mg :: 0.015 g : x mg
$x = 1000 \times 0.015$
$x = 15$

$$\frac{1\text{ g}}{1000\text{ mg}} = \frac{0.015\text{ g}}{x\text{ mg}}$$

$x = 15$

Larger to smaller, so you multiply

1 g = 1000 mg

$0.015 \times 1000 = 15$

$0.015.$

Note: When multiplying in the metric system, move the decimal point to the right. When dividing in the metric system, move the decimal point to the right.

Example 5: gr ss = _____ mg

1 : 60 mg :: gr ½ : x mg
$x = 60 \times \frac{1}{2}$
$x = 30$

$$\frac{\text{gr } 1}{60\text{ mg}} = \frac{\text{gr } \frac{1}{2}}{x\text{ mg}}$$

$x = 30$

Larger to smaller, so you multiply

gr 1 = 60 mg

$$\text{gr } \frac{1}{2} \times 60 = \frac{60}{2} = 30$$

Example 6: 15 mg = gr _____

gr 1 : 60 mg :: gr x : 15 mg

$$\frac{\text{gr } 1}{60\text{ mg}} = \frac{\text{gr } x}{15\text{ mg}}$$

Smaller to larger, so you divide

$60x = 15$

$$\frac{6\cancel{0}x}{6\cancel{0}} = \frac{15}{60}$$

$60x = 15$

$$\frac{6\cancel{0}x}{6\cancel{0}} = \frac{15}{60}$$

gr 1 = 60 mg

$$\frac{15}{60} = \frac{1}{4}$$

$$x = \frac{15}{60} = \frac{1}{4}$$

$$x = \frac{15}{60} = \frac{1}{4}$$

HANDOUT Equivalents

The clock method demonstrates the conversions of common apothecary measurements to milligram measurements. It is based on the equivalent that gr 1 = 60 mg.

There are 60 minutes in an hour. Draw a circle that represents a clock. Write 15, 30, 45, and 60 minutes on the outside of the clock. Erase the words "minutes" and replace them with "milligrams." Fifteen (15) minutes can also be referred to as "quarter past the hour," and 30 minutes can also be referred to as "half past the hour." These fractions are then placed inside the clock. Precede each with the grain symbol. This exercise will help you remember common grain-to-milligram conversions because 15 mg = gr $^1/_4$, 30 mg = gr $^1/_2$.

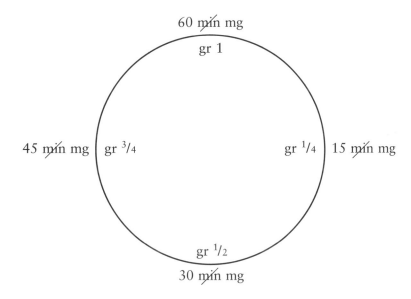

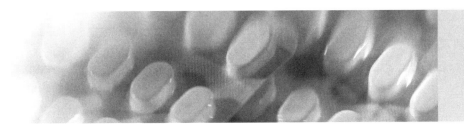

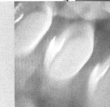

Transparency Originals

1. Solving a Simple Proportion Problem

2. Temperature Conversions

3. Temperature Conversions

4. Example of Times for Administering Medications

5. Conversion of AM-PM Time to Military Time

6. Equivalents

7. Six Rights of Medication Administration

8. Example of Physician's Orders

9. Example of Patient's Medication Administration Record

10. Example of Drug Label (Keflex)

11. Example of Drug Label (Erythromycin)

12. Formula: $\dfrac{D}{A} \times Q = x$

13. Medicine Cup

14. Insulin Syringes

15. Mixed Insulin in Syringes

16. 3 cc, 10 cc, and Tuberculin Syringes

17. Formula: Intravenous Piggyback

18. Formula: Critical Care (mcg/kg/min)

19. Formula: Critical Care (mcg/min)

20. West Nomogram for Body Surface Area Estimation in Children

SOLVING A SIMPLE PROPORTION PROBLEM

1. Multiply the means.

2. Multiply the extremes.

3. Place the product including the x on the *left* and the product of the known terms on the *right*.

4. Divide the product of the known terms by the number next to the x. The quotient will be the value of x.

$$2 : 8 :: 4 : x$$

TEMPERATURE CONVERSIONS

Approximate Equivalents between Celsius and Fahrenheit Measurements

Many hospitals and health care centers use the metric system of measurement, including thermometers calibrated in the Celsius scale. It may be necessary for the nurse to convert the Celsius, or centigrade, scale to the Fahrenheit scale for patient or family information. Because not everyone concerned with patient care uses the same scale, it is also important for the nurse to be able to convert the Fahrenheit scale to the Celsius scale.

Most hospitals now use digital thermometers rather than mercury thermometers. The following thermometers are included for illustration purposes only. Digital thermometers are available in the Fahrenheit or Celsius scale. Patients frequently ask for conversion charts at the time of discharge so that they can understand the readings when they take home their hospital thermometers. The conversion charts are helpful for the nurse as well. However, the nurse should be able to convert from one scale to the other, if necessary.

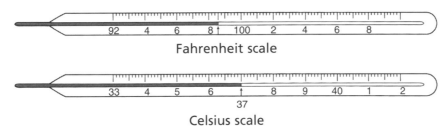

Fahrenheit scale

Celsius scale

For conversion from one scale to another, the following proportion may be used:

Celsius (C) : Fahrenheit (F) − 32 :: 5 : 9
C : F −32 :: 5 : 9

C or F will be the unknown. Extend the decimal to hundredths; round to tenths.

TEMPERATURE CONVERSIONS

Another means of converting Celsius and Fahrenheit temperatures to equivalents is to follow the rules listed in the following box.

CONVERTING CELSIUS AND FAHRENHEIT TEMPERATURES

Fahrenheit to Celsius	*Celsius to Fahrenheit*
Subtract 32	Multiply by 1.8
Divide by 1.8	Add 32

The following examples illustrate each method:

Example: 100.6° F equals _____ ° C.

C : F − 32 :: 5 : 9   100.6 − 32 = 68.6

C : 100.6 − 32 :: 5 : 9   68.6 + 1.8 = 38.111...or 38.1° C

9° C = (100.6° − 32) × 5

9° C = 68.6° × 5

9° C = 343

$$C = \frac{343}{9}$$

C = 38.11

100.6° F = 38.1° C

EXAMPLE OF TIMES FOR ADMINISTERING MEDICATIONS

Abbreviations	Definition	Example Times of Administration
ac*	Before meals	7:30-11:30-5:30
AM	Morning, before noon	9 AM
bid	Twice a day	9-9
hs	At bedtime	9 PM
pc*	After meals	8:30-12:30-6:30
PM	Evening, before midnight	9 PM
prn	As needed	
qd	Once a day	9 AM
qh	Every hour	8-9-10-etc
q2h	Every 2 hours	8-10-12-etc
q3h	Every 3 hours	9-12-3-etc
q4h	Every 4 hours	8-12-4-etc
q6h	Every 6 hours	9-3-9-3
q8h	Every 8 hours	8-4-12
q12h	Every 12 hours	9-9
qid	Four times a day	8-12-4-8
qod	Every other day	
qoh	Every other hour	8-10-12-2-4-6-etc
STAT	Immediately	
tid	Three times a day	9-1-5

*Providing that meals are served at 8:00 AM, 12:00 noon, and 6:00 PM.

CONVERSION OF AM-PM TIME TO MILITARY TIME

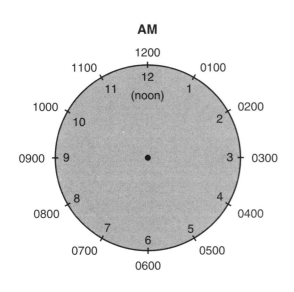

AM

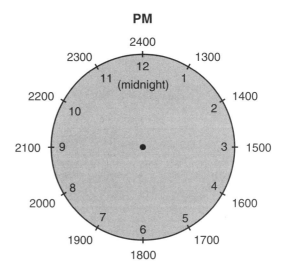

PM

0100-1:00 AM	0900-9:00 AM	1700-5:00 PM
0200-2:00 AM	1000-10:00 AM	1800-6:00 PM
0300-3:00 AM	1100-11:00 AM	1900-7:00 PM
0400-4:00 AM	1200-12:00 noon	2000-8:00 PM
0500-5:00 AM	1300-1:00 PM	2100-9:00 PM
0600-6:00 AM	1400-2:00 PM	2200-10:00 PM
0700-7:00 AM	1500-3:00 PM	2300-11:00 PM
0800-8:00 AM	1600-4:00 PM	2400-12:00 midnight

EQUIVALENTS

Metric Measurements

Weight

   1 kg = 1000 g
   1 g = 1000 mg
   1 g = 1,000,000 mcg
   1 mg = 1000 mcg

Volume

   1 L = 1000 mL
   1 mL = 1 cc

Length

   1 m = 100 cm
   1 m = 1000 mm

Apothecary Measurements

   1 qt = 32 oz = 2 pt
   1 pt = 16 oz
   4 qt = 1 gal

Household Measurements

   1 T = 3 t
   2 T = 1 oz
   1 lb = 16 oz
   1 med glass = 8 oz

Intersystem Measurements

   1 g = gr 15
   gr 1 = 60 mg (65 mg)
   1 t = 5 mL
   1 T = 3 t = 15 mL = $\frac{1}{2}$ oz
   1 oz = 30 mL
   1 L = 1 qt = 32 oz = 2 pt = 4 cups
   1 pt = 500 mL = 16 oz = 2 cups

SIX RIGHTS OF MEDICATION ADMINISTRATION

1. **Drug**

2. **Dose**

3. **Patient**

4. **Route**

5. **Time**

6. **Documentation**

EXAMPLE OF PHYSICIAN'S ORDERS

PHYSICIAN'S ORDERS	Patient, James A.
1. ADDRESSOGRAPH BEFORE PLACING IN PATIENT'S CHART ▶	
2. INITIAL AND DETACH COPY EACH TIME PHYSICIAN WRITES ORDERS	
3. TRANSMIT COPY TO PHARMACY	
4. ORDERS MUST BE DATED AND TIMED	

DATE	ORDERS			TRANS BY
	Diagnosis:	Weight:	Height:	
	Sensitivities/Drug Allergies:			
1/12/07	0900	Lasix 80 mg. p.o. b.i.d.		
		Digoxin 0.125 mg. p.o. q.d.		
		Slow-K 10 mEq. p.o. b.i.d.		
		A. Physician, M.D.		

MEDICAL RECORDS COPY		**PHYSICIAN'S ORDERS**						**T-5**
B-CLIN. NOTES	E-LAB	G-X-RAY	K-DIAGNOSTIC	M-SURGERY	Q-THERAPY	T-ORDERS	W-NURSING	Y-MISC.

Courtesy Clarian Health, Indianapolis, Indiana.

EXAMPLE OF PATIENT'S MEDICATION ADMINISTRATION RECORD

| Transcription of Med Sheet by: _____ | | | | | | | | | | |

Reviewed by: _____   Page _____ of _____

Initials	Signature		Allergies:	☑ NKDA	Injection Sites: A = RUE B = LUE E = Abdomen C = RLE F = R Glut D = LLE G = L Glut	Patient, James A.

Special Notes:

☐ Inpatient   ☐ Outpatient

| *NJ* | *N. Jones R.N.* |
| *AN* | *A. Nurse R. N.* |

See Legend on Back

											DATES					
DATE	DRUG				08 09 10 11	12 13 14 15	16 17 18 19	20 21 22 23	24 01 02 03	04 05 06 07	1/12/07	1/13/07	1/14/07	1/15/07	1/16/07
1 1/12	Lasix										09 AN 21 NJ	09 21 AN NJ			
	80 mg dose	p.o. route	b.i.d. interval	09			21								
2 1/12	Digoxin										09 AN	09 AN			
	0.125 mg dose	p.o. route	q.d. interval	09											
3 1/12	Slow-K										09 AN 21 NJ	09 21 AN NJ			
	10 mEq dose	p.o. route	b.i.d. interval	09			21								
4															
	dose	route	interval												
5															
	dose	route	interval												

MEDICATION PROFILE

B-CLIN. NOTES	E-LAB	G-X-RAY	K-DIAGNOSTIC	M-SURGERY	Q-THERAPY	T-ORDERS	W-NURSING	Y-MISC.

Courtesy Clarian Health, Indianapolis, Indiana.

EXAMPLE OF DRUG LABEL (KEFLEX)

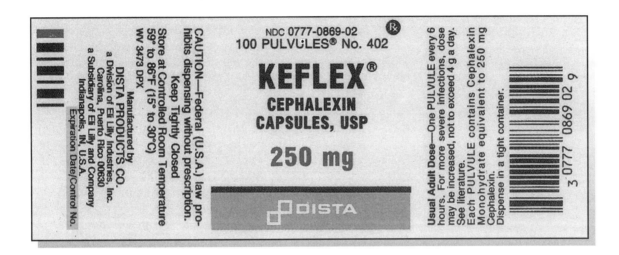

1. Trade name   **Keflex**

2. Generic name   **cephalexin**

3. Dosage strength   **250 mg**

4. Form   **Capsules**

5. Amount   100

6. Directions   **Keep tightly closed. Store at controlled room temperature 59° to 86° F (15° to 30° C).**

7. NDC number   0777-0869-02

8. Manufacturer   **DISTA**

9. Expiration date   **(Highlighted)**

EXAMPLE OF DRUG LABEL (ERYTHROMYCIN)

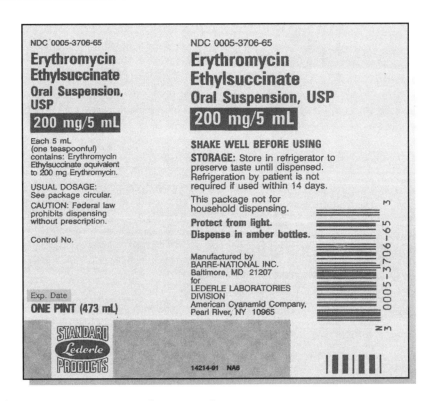

NDC 0005-3706-65

Erythromycin Ethylsuccinate

Oral Suspension, USP

200 mg/5 mL

Each 5 mL (one teaspoonful) contains: Erythromycin Ethylsuccinate equivalent to 200 mg Erythromycin.

USUAL DOSAGE: See package circular.

CAUTION: Federal law prohibits dispensing without prescription.

Control No.

Exp. Date

ONE PINT (473 mL)

STANDARD *Lederle* PRODUCTS

NDC 0005-3706-65

Erythromycin Ethylsuccinate

Oral Suspension, USP

200 mg/5 mL

SHAKE WELL BEFORE USING

STORAGE: Store in refrigerator to preserve taste until dispensed. Refrigeration by patient is not required if used within 14 days.

This package not for household dispensing.

Protect from light.
Dispense in amber bottles.

Manufactured by BARRE-NATIONAL INC. Baltimore, MD 21207 for LEDERLE LABORATORIES DIVISION American Cyanamid Company, Pearl River, NY 10965

0005-3706-65 3

14214-91 NA6

1. Trade name — **Erythromycin**
2. Generic name — **erythromycin ethylsuccinate**
3. Dosage strength — **200 mg/5 mL**
4. Form — **Suspension**
5. Route — **Oral**
6. Amount — **1 pint or 473 mL**
7. Directions — **Shake well before using. Store in refrigerator to preserve taste until dispensed. Refrigeration by patient is not required if used within 14 days. Protect from light. Dispense in amber bottles.**
8. NDC number — **0005-3706-65**
9. Manufacturer — **Barre-National Inc. for Lederle Laboratories Division**
10. Expiration date — **(Highlighted)**

FORMULA

$$\text{Formula: } \frac{D}{A} \times Q = x$$

D Represents the desired amount of the medication that has been ordered by the physician.

A Represents the strength of the medication that is available.

Q Represents the quantity or amount of the medication that contains the available strength.

Note: *When the medication is a solid such as a tablet, capsule, or caplet, the quantity will always be 1. If the medication is in liquid form, the number will vary. Remember from the math review, the denominator of a whole number is always one:* $\frac{1}{1}, \frac{2}{1}, \frac{3}{1}$, *etc.*

x Represents the dosage that is unknown.

This formula can be read as:

> Desired over available multiplied by the quantity available equals *x* or the amount to be given to the patient.

MEDICINE CUP

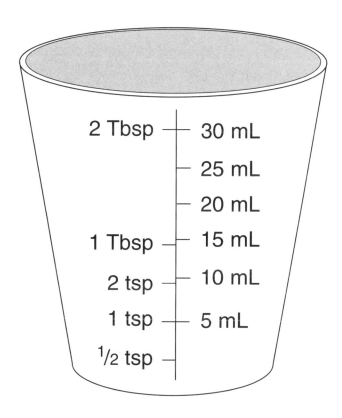

2 Tbsp — 30 mL

— 25 mL

— 20 mL

1 Tbsp — 15 mL

2 tsp — 10 mL

1 tsp — 5 mL

1/2 tsp —

INSULIN SYRINGES

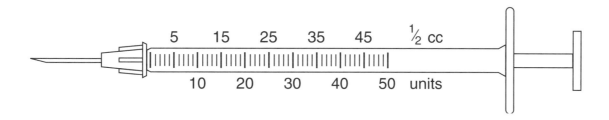

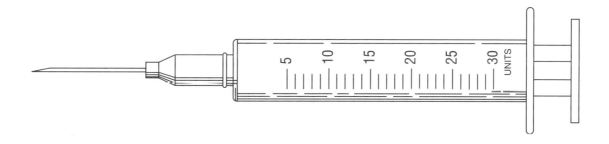

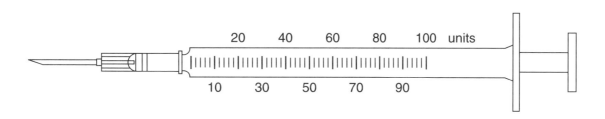

MIXED INSULIN IN SYRINGES

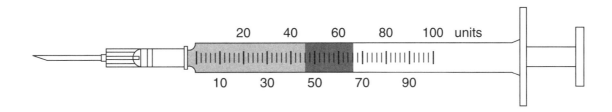

3 CC, 10 CC, AND TUBERCULIN SYRINGES

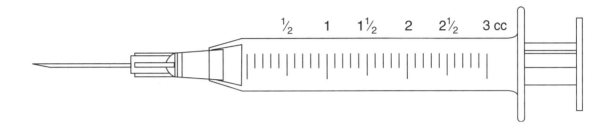

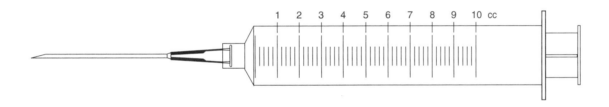

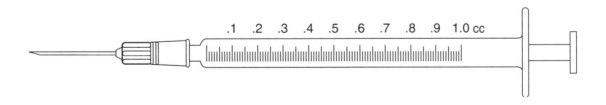

FORMULA: INTRAVENOUS PIGGYBACK

$$\frac{\text{Total volume to be infused}}{\text{Total amount of time in minutes}} \times \text{Drop factor} = x \text{ gtt/min}$$

$$\frac{V}{T} \times C = R$$

When the volume, time, or length of infusion and the constant drip factor are known, a simple formula may be used.

$$\frac{V \text{ (volume)}}{T \text{ (time)}} \times C \text{ (constant drip factor)} = R \text{ (gtt/min)}$$

FORMULA: CRITICAL CARE (MCG/KG/MIN)

The formula for calculating the mL/hr is:

$$\frac{\text{Ordered mcg/kg/min} \times \text{Patient's weight in kg} \times 60 \text{ min/1 hr*}}{\text{Medication concentration (\# of mcg/1 mL)}}$$

*60 min/1 hr is a constant fraction in the formula and represents the equivalency of 60 minutes = 1 hour.

FORMULA: CRITICAL CARE (MCG/MIN)

The formula is:

$$\frac{\text{Ordered mcg/min} \times 60 \text{ min/1 hr*}}{\text{Medication concentration (\# of mcg/mL)}}$$

*60 min/1 hr is a constant fraction in the formula and represents the equivalency of 60 minutes = 1 hour.

WEST NOMOGRAM FOR BODY SURFACE AREA ESTIMATION IN CHILDREN

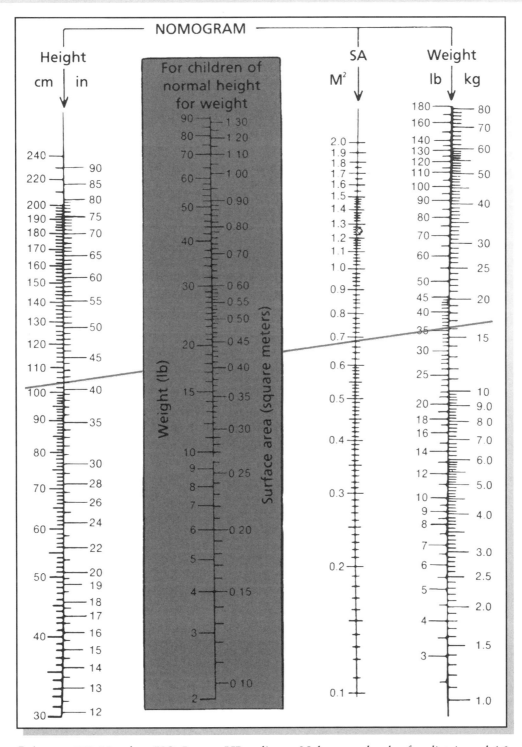

NOMOGRAM

Height		For children of normal height for weight	SA	Weight
cm	in	Weight (lb) / Surface area (square meters)	M²	lb	kg

From Behrman RE, Vaughan VC, Jenson HB, editors: *Nelson textbook of pediatrics,* ed 16, Philadelphia, 2000, WB Saunders; modified from data of E Boyd by CD West.

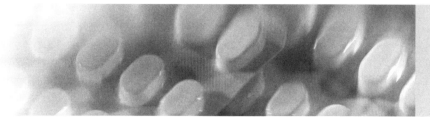

Test Bank

FRACTIONS

Directions: Perform the indicated calculations, and reduce the fraction to the lowest terms.

1. $^5/_8 + 3^1/_6 =$ _____

2. $5^1/_9 - 3^2/_3 =$ _____

3. $1^5/_7 - ^4/_5 =$ _____

4. $7^1/_2 \times 5^2/_3 =$ _____

5. $^3/_{10} \div 2 =$ _____

6. $^6/_7 / 1^1/_3 =$ _____

DECIMALS

Directions: Perform the indicated calculations, and reduce fractions to the lowest terms.

7. $2.43 + 140.59 + 839.78 + 0.999 =$ _____

8. $20.48 - 8.79 =$ _____

9. $0.76 \times 0.08 =$ _____

10. $8.053 \times 0.024 =$ _____

11. $216.48 \div 55 =$ _____

12. $248 \div 0.008 =$ _____

PERCENTS

13. Change $^7/_{30}$ to a percent: _____

14. Change 0.3276 to a percent: _____

15. Change 58% to a proper fraction: _____

16. Change 2.93% to a decimal: _____

17. What percent of 325 is 75? _____

18. What is 3.5% of 57? _____

RATIOS

19. Change $^3/_8$ / $^1/_4$ to a ratio reduced to its lowest terms: _____

20. Change 0.756 to a ratio reduced to its lowest terms: _____

21. Change 35% to a ratio reduced to its lowest terms: _____

22. Change $^4/_7$: $^2/_5$ to a fraction reduced to its lowest terms: _____

23. Change 20 : 32 to a decimal number: _____

24. Change $^3/_{25}$: $^4/_{75}$ to a percent: _____

PROPORTIONS

Directions: Find the value of x.

25. $^1/_{300}$: 4 :: 6 : x: _____

26. 24 : x :: 6 : 60: _____

27. 9 : x :: 3 : 800: _____

28. 15 : 16 :: 120 : x: _____

29. x : 12 :: 9 : 6: _____

30. 6 : 20 :: x : 120: _____

31. 0.6 : x :: 0.4 : 12: _____

32. 83.25 : 60 :: x : 45: _____

METRIC AND HOUSEHOLD MEASUREMENTS

Directions: Change to the designated equivalents.

33. 18 mg = _____ mcg

34. 280 mcg = _____ g

35. 3 kg = _____ g

36. 7 cm = _____ mm

37. 0.54 L = _____ mL

38. 4.7 lb = _____ g

APOTHECARY AND HOUSEHOLD MEASUREMENTS

Directions: Change to the approximate equivalent.

39. 5 gal = _____ qt

40. 2 coffee cups = _____ fl oz

41. 3 qt = _____ fl oz

42. 20 fl oz = _____ pt

EQUIVALENTS BETWEEN APOTHECARY AND METRIC MEASUREMENTS

Directions: Change to approximate equivalents as indicated.

43. 320 mL = _____ fl oz

44. 4 gr = _____ g

45. 75 mg = _____ gr

46. 1.4 L = _____ qt

47. 115 lb = _____ kg

48. $^1/_{10}$ gr = _____ mg

49. 39.7° C = _____ ° F

50. 96.4° F = _____ ° C

DIMENSIONAL ANALYSIS AND THE CALCULATION OF DRUG DOSAGES

51. The physician has ordered Pravachol 40 mg po daily for control of high cholesterol. The medication is supplied in 20 mg tablets. How many tablets will the nurse administer?

_____

52. The physician has ordered Wellbutrin 75 mg po for smoking cessation. The medication is supplied in 150 mg tablets. How many tablets will the nurse administer?

_____

53. The physician has ordered Demerol 50 mg IM q4h for pain. The medication is supplied in Demerol 100 mg in 1 mL. How many milliliters will the nurse administer?

_____

54. The physician has ordered Benadryl 75 mg IM for a rash. The medication is supplied in Benadryl 50 mg in 1 mL. How many tablets will the nurse administer?

_____

55. The physician has ordered penicillin G procaine 1.2 millionunits IM for infection. The medication is supplied in 600,000 millionunits in 1 mL. How many milliliters will the nurse administer?

_____

56. The physician has ordered heparin 7500 units subcutaneous (SQ) daily. The medication is supplied in heparin 10,000 units in 1 mL. How many milliliters will the nurse administer?

_____

57. The physician has ordered Pitocin 20 units IM immediately (stat). The medication is supplied in Pitocin 10 units in 1 mL. How many milliliters will the nurse administer?

_____

58. The physician has ordered gentamycin 80 mg IVPB every 12 hours for infection. The medication is supplied in gentamycin 80 mg in 100 mL to infuse over 1 hour (tubing: 15 gtts/mL). How many gtts/min will be given?

   _____

59. The physician has ordered an IV of 1000 mL D$_5$0.45% normal saline (NS) to infuse over 8 hours. Tubing drop factor is 20 gtts/mL. How many milliliters will the nurse administer?

   _____

60. The physician has ordered a continuous heparin drip at 1000 units per hour for pulmonary embolus. The IV is supplied in 25,000 units heparin in 500 mL D$_5$W. How many mL/hr will the pump be programmed for?

   _____

ORAL DOSAGES

61. The physician has ordered Methergine 0.4 mg po bid for postpartum bleeding. The medication is supplied in 0.2 mg tablets. How many tablets will the nurse administer?

   _____

62. The physician has ordered Synthroid 150 mcg po qd for hypothyroidism. The medication is supplied in 0.15 mg/tablet. How many tablets will the nurse administer?

   _____

63. The physician has ordered Paxil 30 mg po qd for depression. The medication is supplied in 10 mg tablets. How many tablets will the nurse administer?

   _____

64. The physician has ordered Seconal 300 mg po prn for sleep. The medication is supplied in 100 mg capsules. How many capsules will the nurse administer?

   _____

65. The physician has ordered acyclovir 200 mg po tid for herpes. The medication is supplied in 200 mg tablets. How many tablets will the nurse administer?

_____

66. The physician has ordered Salagen 2.5 mg po bid for dry eyes. The medication is supplied in 5 mg tablets. How many tablets will the nurse administer?

_____

67. The physician has ordered ASA 650 mg po every 4 to 6 hours for temperature higher than 101° F. The medication is supplied in gr v tablets. How many tablets will the nurse administer?

_____

68. The physician has ordered Cipro 500 mg po bid for sinusitis. The medication is supplied in 250 mg tablets. How many tablets will the nurse administer?

_____

69. The physician has ordered Lanoxin elixir 90 mcg po daily for congestive heart failure. How many milliliters will the nurse administer?

_____

60 mL   NDC 0173-0264-27

LANOXIN®
(DIGOXIN)
ELIXIR
PEDIATRIC
Each mL contains
50 μg (0.05 mg)
PLEASANTLY FLAVORED

GlaxoWellcome
Glaxo Wellcome Inc.
Research Triangle Park, NC 27709
Made in U.S.A.   Rev. 2/96   542404

Alcohol 10%, Methylparaben 0.1%
(added as a preservative)
For indications, dosage, precautions, etc.,
see accompanying package insert.
Store at 15° to 25°C (59° to 77°F) and
protect from light.
CAUTION: Federal law prohibits
dispensing without prescription.

LOT
EXP

70. The physician has ordered KCL 30 mEq po daily for hypokalemia. The medication is supplied in 40 mEq/15 mL. How many milliliters will the nurse administer?

_____

71. The physician has ordered Benadryl elixir 25 mg po for hives. How many milliliters will the nurse administer?

_____

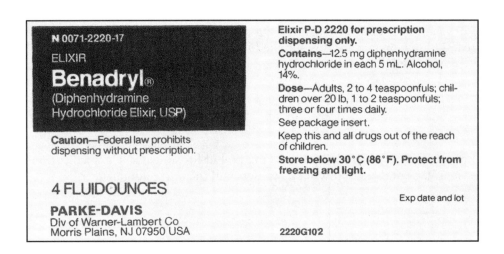

N 0071-2220-17

ELIXIR

Benadryl®

(Diphenhydramine
Hydrochloride Elixir, USP)

Caution—Federal law prohibits
dispensing without prescription.

4 FLUIDOUNCES

PARKE-DAVIS
Div of Warner-Lambert Co
Morris Plains, NJ 07950 USA

**Elixir P-D 2220 for prescription
dispensing only.**

Contains—12.5 mg diphenhydramine
hydrochloride in each 5 mL. Alcohol,
14%.

Dose—Adults, 2 to 4 teaspoonfuls; children over 20 lb, 1 to 2 teaspoonfuls;
three or four times daily.

See package insert.

Keep this and all drugs out of the reach
of children.

**Store below 30°C (86°F). Protect from
freezing and light.**

Exp date and lot

2220G102

72. The physician has ordered Zantac elixir 75 mg po bid for heartburn. The medication is supplied in 15 mg/mL. How many milliliters will the nurse administer? Shade the medicine cup to indicate the correct dosage.

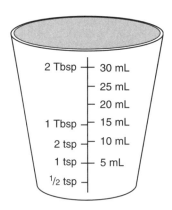

2 Tbsp —— 30 mL
              —— 25 mL
              —— 20 mL
1 Tbsp —— 15 mL
2 tsp —— 10 mL
1 tsp —— 5 mL
½ tsp ——

73. The physician has ordered Dilantin oral suspension 100 mg po tid for seizures. The medication is supplied in 125 mg/5 mL. How many milliliters will the nurse administer? Shade the syringe to indicate the correct dose.

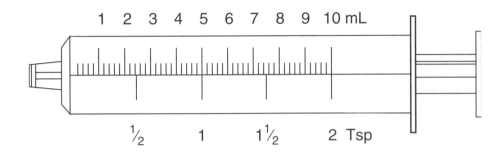

74. The physician has ordered Prozac liquid 40 mg po daily for depression. How many milliliters will the nurse administer?

_____

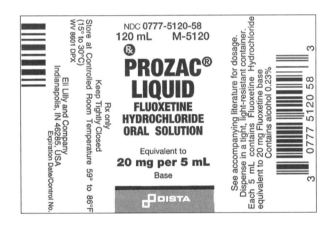

75. The physician has ordered nitroglycerin tablets gr $^1/_{200}$ sublingual every 5 minutes up to 3 tablets for chest pain. The medication is supplied in 0.3 mg tablets. The patient took 3 tablets. How many mg did she receive?

_____

PARENTERAL DOSAGES

76. The physician has ordered Reconbivax 5 mcg IM for hepatitis B vaccination. The medication is supplied in 5 mcg/0.5 mL. How many milliliters will the nurse administer? Shade the syringe.

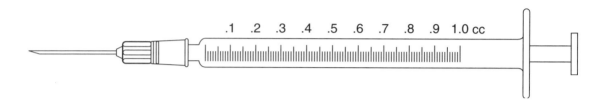

77. The physician has ordered Methergine 0.2 mg IM for postpartum bleeding. The medication is supplied in 0.2 mg/mL. How many milliliters will the nurse administer? Shade the syringe.

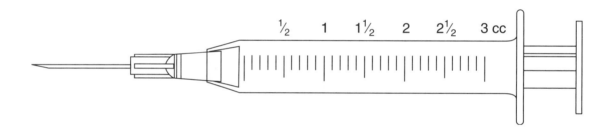

78. The physician has ordered Stadol 3 mg IM for pain. The medication is supplied in 1 mg/mL. How many milliliters will the nurse administer? Shade the syringe.

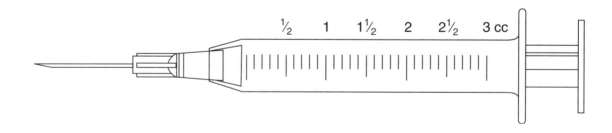

79. The physician has ordered Toradol 60 mg IM for migraine headache. The medication is supplied in 30 mg/mL. How many milliliters will the nurse administer? Shade the syringe.

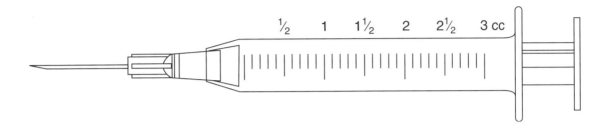

80. The physician has ordered Lovenox 40 mg SQ qd for prevention of deep venous thrombosis (DVT). The medication is supplied in 40 mg/0.4 mL. How many milliliters will the nurse administer? Shade the syringe.

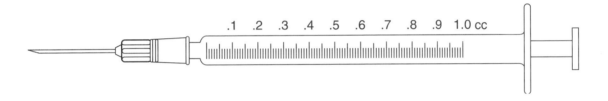

81. The physician has ordered testosterone 150 mg IM weekly for hormone replacement. The medication is supplied in 200 mg/mL. How many milliliters will the nurse administer? Shade the syringe.

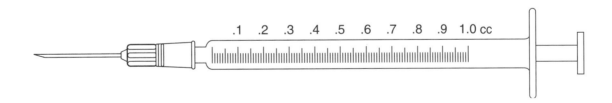

82. The physician has ordered Neupogen 360 mcg SQ qd for neutropenia. The medication is supplied in 300 mcg/mL. How many milliliters will the nurse administer? Shade the syringe.

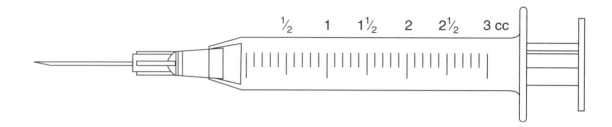

83. The physician has ordered furosemide 20 mg IM stat for edema. How many milliliters will the nurse administer?

_____

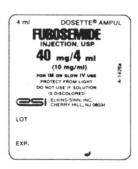

84. The physician has ordered KCL 20 mEq in 1000 D$_5$ NS to infuse at 100 mL/hr. How many milliliters will the nurse add to the IV?

_____

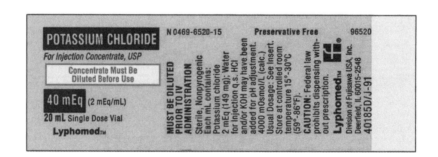

85. The physician has ordered Imitrex 6 mg SQ for migraine headache. The medication is supplied in 12 mg/mL. How many milliliters will the nurse administer?

_____

86. The physician has ordered Imferon 75 mg IM (Z track) for anemia. The medication is supplied in 50 mg/mL. How many milliliters will the nurse administer?

_____

87. The physician has ordered Solu-Cortef 125 mg IM q8h. How many milliliters will the nurse administer?

_____

Single-Dose Vial   For IV or IM use
Contains Benzyl Alcohol as a Preservative
See package insert for complete
product information.
Per 2 mL (when mixed):
* hydrocortisone sodium succinate equiv.
to hydrocortisone, 250 mg. Protect
solution from light. Discard after 3 days.
814 070 205   Reconstituted . . . .
The Upjohn Company
Kalamazoo, MI 49001, USA

2 mL Act-O-Vial®   NDC 0009-0909-08
Solu-Cortef®   Sterile Powder
hydrocortisone sodium succinate
for injection, USP
250 mg*

88. The physician has ordered morphine 12 mg IM every 4 to 6 hours for pain. How many milliliters will the nurse administer?

_____

NDC 0002-1637-01
20 mL   VIAL No. 336
POISON Lilly C II
MORPHINE
SULFATE   15
INJECTION, USP
15 mg per mL
Multiple Dose

APPROXIMATE VOLUME SCALE
—20
—15
—10
—5

APPROXIMATE EQUIVALENTS
0.5 mL   8 mg
0.7 mL   10 mg
1 mL   15 mg

89. The physician has ordered 20 mg of medication diluted in 100 mL D$_5$W given over 15 to 30 minutes IV. The medication is supplied in 40 mg/5 mL. How many milliliters will the nurse add to the IV solution?

_____

90. The physician has ordered Atropine 0.3 mg IM preoperatively. How many milliliters will the nurse administer?

_____

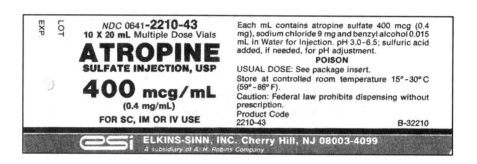

DOSAGES MEASURED IN UNITS

91. The physician has ordered heparin 6500 units SQ for DVT prevention. The medication is supplied in 10,000 units/mL. How many milliliters will the nurse administer?

_____

92. The physician has ordered heparin 7000 units SQ qd postoperatively. The medication is supplied in 5000 units/mL. How many milliliters will the nurse administer? Shade the syringe.

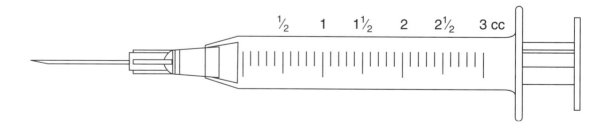

93. The physician has ordered penicillin G procaine 4.8 million units IM for gonorrhea to be given in two injections. Each injection should be 2.4 million units. The medication is supplied in 1.2 million units/2 mL. How many milliliters will the nurse administer? Shade the syringe.

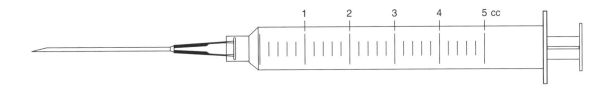

94. The physician has ordered Epogen 5400 units SQ for red blood cell (RBC) production. The medication is supplied in 4000 units/mL. How many milliliters will the nurse administer? Shade the syringe.

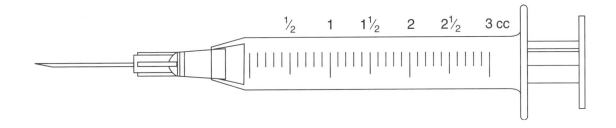

95. The physician has ordered Humulin R (regular) insulin 12 units SQ every morning. How many milliliters will the nurse administer? Shade the syringe.

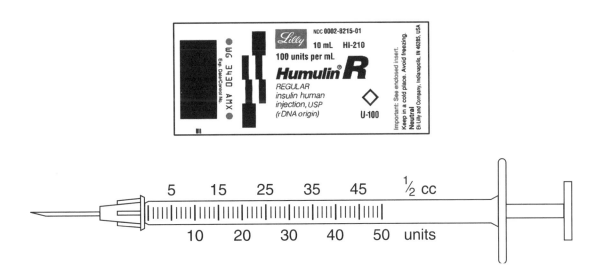

96. The physician has ordered insulin lispro 4 units SQ. The medication is supplied in 100 units/mL. How many milliliters will the nurse administer? Shade the syringe.

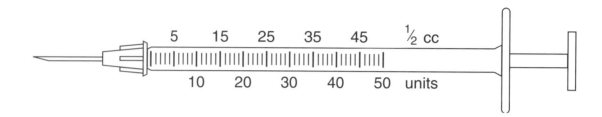

97. The physician has ordered Humulin NPH (neutral protamine hagedorn) insulin 22 units plus Humulin R insulin 12 units SQ every evening. The medication is supplied in 100 units/mL. How many milliliters will the nurse administer? Shade the syringe.

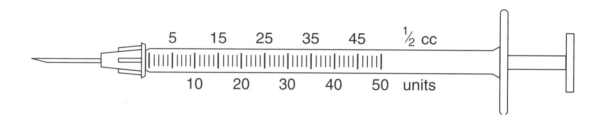

98. The physician has ordered Humulin NPH insulin 38 units plus Humulin R insulin 16 units SQ every morning. The medication is supplied in 100 units/mL. How many milliliters will the nurse administer? Shade the syringe.

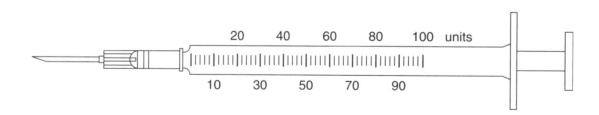

99. The physician has ordered Humulin NPH insulin 50 units plus Humulin R insulin 22 units SQ every afternoon. The medication is supplied in 100 units/mL. How many milliliters will the nurse administer? Shade the syringe.

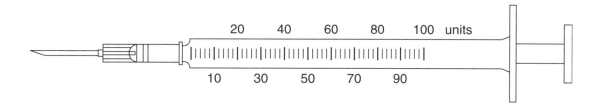

100. The physician has ordered Humulin NPH insulin 44 units plus Humulin R insulin 15 units SQ every morning. The medication is supplied in 100 units/mL. How many milliliters will the nurse administer? Shade the syringe.

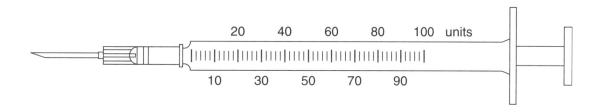

INTRAVENOUS FLOW RATES

101. The physician has ordered magnesium sulfate 1 g qd. The medication is supplied in 4 g/250 mL. Calculate the flow rate in mL/hr.

    _____

102. The physician has ordered to infuse 1 L in 10 hours. Calculate the flow rate in mL/hr.

    _____

103. The physician has ordered Pepcid 20 mg IVPB every 12 hours. The medication is supplied in 20 mg/100 mL to infuse over 20 minutes. Calculate the flow rate in mL/hr.

    _____

104. The physician has ordered a continuous IV Dilaudid drip at 1 mg/hr. The medication is supplied in 20 mg/100 mL. Calculate the flow rate in mL/hr.

_____

105. The physician has ordered a continuous IV morphine drip to infuse at 4 mg/hr. The medication is supplied in 50 mg/50 mL. Calculate the flow rate in mL/hr.

_____

106. The physician has ordered to infuse 1 unit (250 mL) of packed red blood cells (PRBC) over 3 hours. Calculate the flow rate in mL/hr.

_____

107. The physician has ordered an IV of 40 mEq in 500 mL 0.9% NS to infuse over 5 hours. Calculate the flow rate in mL/hr.

_____

108. The physician has ordered erythromycin 200 mg in 250 mL of D_5W to infuse in 1 hour. Calculate the flow rate in mL/hr.

_____

109. The physician has ordered to infuse 1000 mL 0.9% NS at 150 mL/hr for dehydration. Calculate the flow rate in gtts/min (tubing: 10 gtts/mL).

_____

110. The physician has ordered 1000 mL lactated Ringers (LR) to infuse at 125 mL/hr for a postoperative patient. Calculate the flow rate in gtts/min (tubing: 15 gtts/mL).

_____

111. The physician has ordered 500 mL NS to infuse at 150 mL/hr for a patient with vomiting. Calculate the flow rate in gtts/min (tubing: 15 gtts/mL).

_____

112. The physician has ordered 1000 mL 0.45% NS to infuse at 60 mL/hr. Calculate the flow rate in gtts/min (tubing: 20 gtts/mL).

_____

113. The physician has ordered vancomycin 500 mg in 250 mL of D_5W IVPB daily to infuse over 2 hours. Calculate the flow rate in gtts/min (tubing: 10 gtts/mL).

_____

114. The physician has ordered ampicillin 1 g in 100 mL of D_5W IVPB to infuse over 45 minutes. Calculate the flow rate in gtts/min (tubing: 60 gtts/mL).

_____

115. The physician has ordered Kefzol 2 g in 50 mL NS IVPB to infuse over 30 minutes. Calculate the flow rate in gtts/min (tubing: 20 gtts/mL).

_____

CRITICAL CARE IV FLOW RATES

116. The physician has ordered to infuse Pitocin IV drip at 0.9 units per hour. The medication is supplied in 15 units/250 mL D_5W. Calculate the flow rate in mL/hr.

_____

117. The physician has ordered to infuse Pitocin IV drip at 0.72 units per hour. The medication is supplied in 30 units/500 mL D_5W. Calculate the flow rate in mL/hr.

_____

118. The physician has ordered heparin IV drip at 1800 units per hour. The medication is supplied in 50,000 units/500 mL D_5W. Calculate the flow rate in mL/hr.

_____

119. The physician has ordered heparin IV drip at 1200 units per hour. The medication is supplied in 25,000 units/500 mL of NS. Calculate the flow rate in mL/hr.

_____

120. The physician has ordered Humulin R insulin IV drip at 6 units per hour. The medication is supplied in 100 units/100 mL of NS. Calculate the flow rate in mL/hr.

_____

121. The physician has ordered Humulin R insulin IV drip at 12 units per hour. The medication is supplied in 50 units/100 mL NS. Calculate the flow rate in mL/hr.

_____

122. The physician has ordered magnesium sulfate IV drip at 2 g/hr for PIH. The medication is supplied in magnesium sulfate 25 g/500 mL D_5W. Calculate the flow rate in mL/hr.

_____

123. The physician has ordered amiodarone IV drip at 1.5 mg/min for ventricular dysrhythmias. The medication is supplied in 900 mg/500 mL of D_5W. Calculate the flow rate in mL/hr.

_____

124. The physician has ordered a lidocaine IV drip to infuse at 4 mg/min for premature ventricular contractions (PVCs). The medication is supplied in 2 g/500 mL of D_5W. Calculate the flow rate in mL/hr.

_____

125. The physician has ordered a nitroglycerin IV drip to infuse at 5 mcg/min for chest pain. The medication is supplied in 25 mg/250 mL of D_5W. Calculate the flow rate in mL/hr.

_____

126. The physician has ordered a Levophed IV drip at 2 mcg/min for hypotension. The medication is supplied in 4 mg/500 mL of D_5W. Calculate the flow rate in mL/hr.

_____

127. The physician has ordered terbutaline IV drip at 10 mcg/min for premature labor. The medication is supplied in 5 mg/500 mL of NS. Calculate the flow rate in mL/hr.

_____

128. The physician has ordered dopamine IV drip at 3 mcg/kg/min for low blood pressure (BP) (weight: 132 pounds). The medication is supplied in 400 mg/250 mL of 0.45% NS. Calculate the flow rate in mL/hr.

_____

129. The physician has ordered esmolol IV drip at 50 mcg/kg/min for tachycardia (weight: 154 pounds). The medication is supplied in 5 g/500 mL of D_5W. Calculate the flow rate in mL/hr.

_____

130. The physician has ordered Nipride IV drip at 3 mcg/kg/min for elevated BP (weight: 176 pounds). The medication is supplied in 50 mg/250 mL of D_5W. Calculate the flow rate in mL/hr.

_____

PEDIATRIC DOSAGES

131. The recommended safe dose for a child of erythromycin is 20 mg/kg/day in four equal doses (weight: 22 pounds). The medication is supplied in 125 mg/mL.

a. Calculate the weight for this child. _____

b. Calculate the safe dose for this child. _____

c. How many milliliters will be administered for each dose? _____

132. The recommended safe dose for a child of rifampin is 5 mg/kg/dose (weight: 10 pounds). The medication is supplied in 10 mg/mL.

a. Calculate the weight for this child. _____

b. Calculate the safe dose for this child. _____

c. How many milliliters will be administered for each dose? _____

133. The recommended dose for a child of oxacillin is 50 mg/kg/day in four equal doses (weight: 46 pounds). The medication is supplied in 250 mg/5 mL.

a. Calculate the weight for this child. _____

b. Calculate the safe dose for this child. _____

c. How many milliliters will be administered for each dose? _____

134. The recommended dose of Lasix for a child is 1 mg/kg/dose (weight: 55 pounds). The medication is supplied in 10 mg/mL.

a. Calculate the weight for this child. _____

b. Calculate the safe dose for this child. _____

c. How many milliliters will be administered for each dose? _____

135. The recommended dose of Tempra for a child 1 to 2 years old is 120 mg every 4 to 6 hours. The medication is supplied in 80 mg/chewable tablet. How many tablets would a 2-year-old child receive?

_____

136. The recommended dose of Dilantin for a child is 7 mg/kg/24 hours given every 12 hours (weight: 44 pounds). The medication is supplied in 125 mg/5 mL.

a. Calculate the weight for this child. _____

b. Calculate the safe dose for this child. _____

c. How many milliliters will be administered for each dose? _____

137. A health care provider ordered 500 mL of D_5 0.45% NS to infuse at 75 mL/hr (tubing: 20 gtts/mL). Calculate the rate in gtts/min.

_____

138. The recommended dose of gentamicin IVPB for a child is 6 mg/kg/day in three equal doses (weight: 55 pounds; tubing: 60 gtts/mL). The medication is supplied in 50 mg/100 mL to infuse over 2 hours.

   a. Calculate the weight for this child. _____

   b. Calculate the dose for this child. _____

   c. Calculate the rate in mL/hr for this IV. _____

   d. Calculate the gtts/min. _____

139. The recommended dose of morphine IV for a child is 0.6 mg/kg/hr (weight: 66 pounds). The medication is supplied in 30 mg/30 mL.

   a. Calculate the weight for this child. _____

   b. Calculate the dose for this child. _____

   c. Calculate the rate in mL/hr for this IV. _____

140. The recommended dose of Zinacef IVPB for a child is 75 mg/kg/day in three equal doses (weight: 88 pounds; tubing: 60 gtts/mL). The medication is supplied in 1000 mg/50 mL to infuse over 30 minutes.

   a. Calculate the weight for this child. _____

   b. Calculate the dose for this child. _____

   c. Calculate the rate in mL/hr for this IV. _____

   d. Calculate the gtts/min. _____

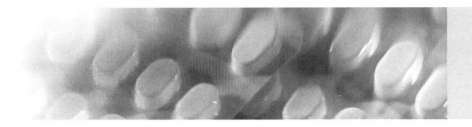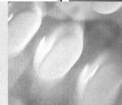

Test Bank Answers

FRACTIONS

1. $3\frac{19}{24}$
2. $1\frac{4}{9}$
3. $\frac{32}{35}$
4. $42\frac{1}{2}$
5. $\frac{3}{20}$
6. $\frac{9}{14}$

DECIMALS

7. 983.799
8. 11.69
9. 0.0608
10. 0.193272
11. 3.936
12. 31,000.0

PERCENTS

13. $23\frac{1}{3}\%$
14. 32.76%
15. $\frac{29}{50}$
16. 0.0293
17. $23\frac{1}{13}\%$ or 23.0769%
18. 1.995

RATIOS

19. 3 : 2
20. 189 : 250
21. 7 : 20
22. $1\frac{3}{7}$
23. 0.625
24. 225%

PROPORTIONS

25. 7200
26. 240
27. 2400
28. 128
29. 18

30. 36
31. 18
32. 62.4375

METRIC AND HOUSEHOLD MEASUREMENTS

33. 18,000 mcg
34. 0.00028 g
35. 3000 g
36. 70 mm
37. 540 mL
38. 2136.36 g

APOTHECARY AND HOUSEHOLD MEASUREMENTS

39. 20 qt
40. 12 fl oz
41. 96 fl oz
42. $1^{1}/_{4}$ pt

EQUIVALENTS BETWEEN APOTHECARY AND METRIC MEASUREMENTS

43. $10^{2}/_{3}$ fl oz
44. 0.2667 g
45. $1^{1}/_{4}$ gr
46. $1^{2}/_{5}$ qt
47. 52.27 kg
48. 6 mg
49. 103.46° F
50. 35.78° C

DIMENSIONAL ANALYSIS AND THE CALCULATION OF DRUG DOSAGES

51. 2 tablets
52. $^{1}/_{2}$ tablet
53. 0.5 mL
54. 1.5 mL
55. 2 mL
56. 0.75 mL
57. 2 mL
58. 25 gtts/min
59. 41 gtts/min
60. 20 mL/hr

ORAL DOSAGES

61. 2 tablets
62. 1 tablet
63. 3 tablets
64. 3 capsules
65. 1 tablet

66. ¹/₂ tablets
67. 2 tablets
68. 2 tablets
69. 1.8 mL
70. 11.25 mL
71. 10 mL
72. 5 mL

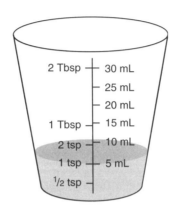

73. 4 mL

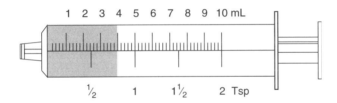

74. 10 mL
75. 0.9 mg

PARENTERAL DOSAGES

76. 0.5 mL

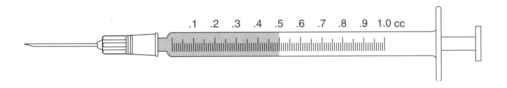

77. 1 mL

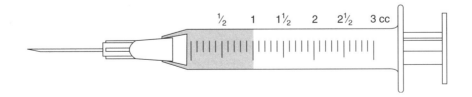

78. 3 mL

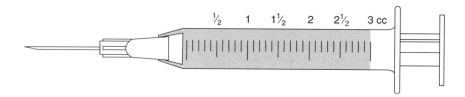

79. 2 mL

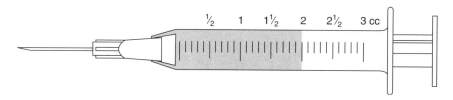

80. 0.4 mL

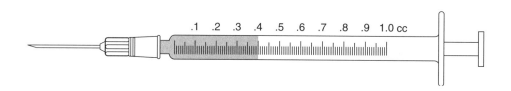

81. 0.75 mL

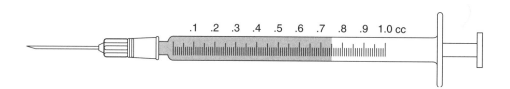

82. 1.2 mL

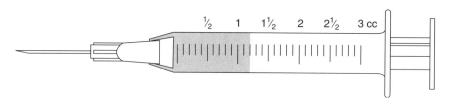

83. 2 mL
84. 10 mL
85. 0.5 mL
86. 1.5 mL
87. 1 mL
88. 0.8 mL
89. 2.5 mL
90. 0.75 mL

DOSAGES MEASURED IN UNITS

91. 0.65 mL
92. 1.4 mL

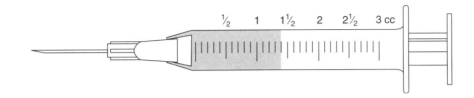

93. 4 mL

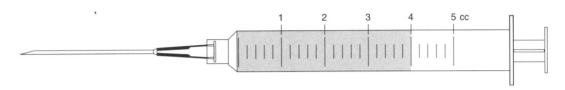

94. 1.4 mL

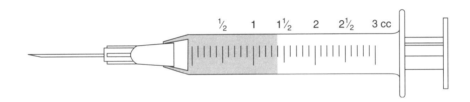

95. 12 units

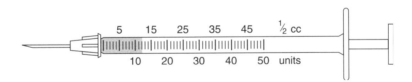

96. 4 units

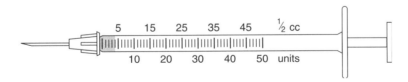

97. Total 34 units

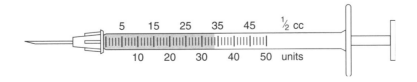

98. Total 54 units

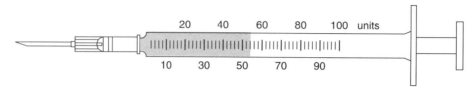

99. Total 72 units

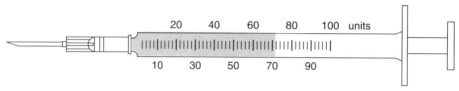

100. Total 59 units

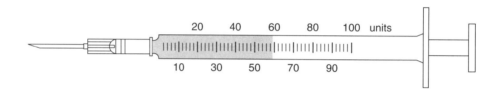

INTRAVENOUS FLOW RATES

101. 63 mL/hr
102. 100 mL/hr
103. 300 mL/hr
104. 5 mL/hr
105. 4 mL/hr
106. 83 mL/hr
107. 100 mL/hr
108. 250 mL/hr
109. 25 gtts/min
110. 31-32 gtts/min
111. 38 gtts/min
112. 20 gtts/min
113. 21 gtts/min
114. 133-134 gtts/min
115. 33-34 gtts/min

CRITICAL CARE IV FLOW RATES

116. 15 mL/hr
117. 12 mL/hr
118. 18 mL/hr
119. 24 mL/hr
120. 6 mL/hr
121. 24 mL/hr
122. 40 mL/hr
123. 50 mL/hr

124. 60 mL/hr
125. 3 mL/hr
126. 15 mL/hr
127. 60 mL/hr
128. 7 mL/hr
129. 21 mL/hr
130. 72 mL/hr

PEDIATRIC DOSAGES

131. a. 10 kg
     b. 50 mg/dose
     c. 0.4 mL/dose
132. a. 4.5 kg
     b. 22.5 mg/dose
     c. 2.25 dose/dose
133. a. 21 kg
     b. 263 mg/dose
     c. 5.2 dose/dose
134. a. 25 kg
     b. 25 mg/dose
     c. 2.5 dose/dose
135. 1.5 tablets
136. a. 20 kg
     b. 70 mg/dose
     c. 2.8 mL/dose
137. 25 gtts/min
138. a. 25 kg
     b. 50 mg/dose
     c. 50 mL/hr
     d. 50 gtts/min
139. a. 30 kg
     b. 18 mg/hr
     c. 18 mL/hr
140. a. 40 kg
     b. 1000 mg/dose
     c. 100 mL/hr
     d. 100 gtts/min